The Simple Keto Slow Cooker Cookbook for Beginners

The complete cookbook for your slow cooker to speed up your metabolism, lower cholesterol and lose weight fast with low carb dishes.

Linda Walker

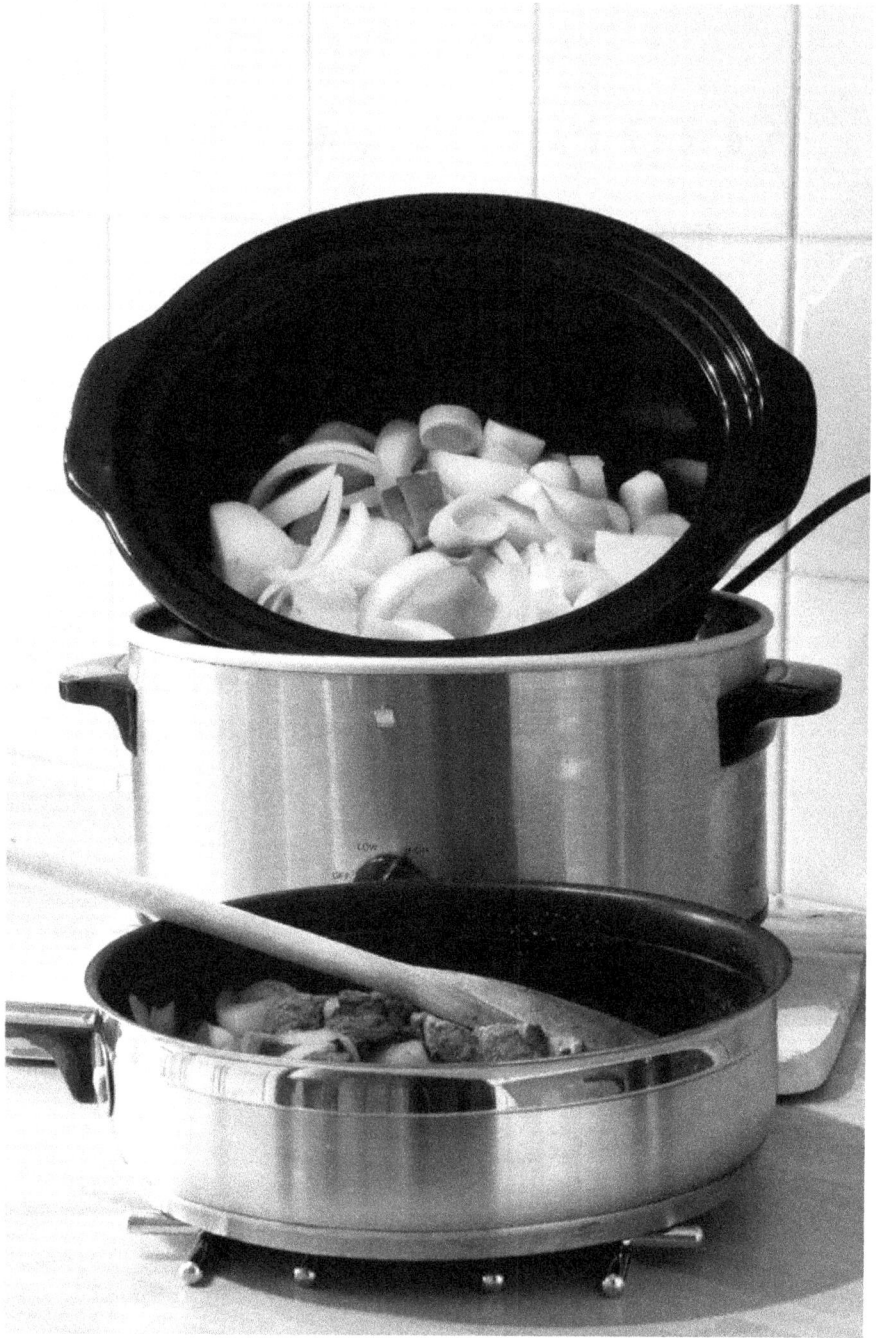

The information in the following pages is broadly considered a truthful and accurate account of facts and as such, any inattention, use, or misuse of the information in question by the reader will render any resulting actions solely under their purview. There are no scenarios in which the publisher or the original author of this work can be in any fashion deemed liable for any hardship or damages that may befall them after undertaking information described herein.

Additionally, the information in the following pages is intended only for informational purposes and should thus be thought of as universal. As befitting its nature, it is presented without assurance regarding its prolonged validity or interim quality. Trademarks that are mentioned are done without written consent and can in no way be considered an endorsement from the trademark holder.

Table of Contents

Introduction

Slow cookers can be really useful in the kitchen and can make life so much easier. They make it so that you can prep your ingredients the day before, and they will be ready for you when you get home. The slow cooker is also great for people on a tight budget, because it can save you a lot of money in the long run. That said, it's important to know how to use your slow cooker properly. Here are some tips to help you get started.

Cook With Low Heat

Always start with low heat when cooking your ingredients in a slow cooker. If you put them over medium heat, they will burn or scorch before they are finished. Instead, start out on low heat and let them cook for several hours until they are done. This will ensure that they are safe to eat and don't have any nasty flavors left over from being cooked too fast.

Leave room at the top

Place your ingredients in the cooker as soon as possible after placing them on the stove top or in the oven. This will give them enough time to cook properly without being overcooked on high heat. If you leave them sitting in the hot pot without food inside of it, sometimes it can become stuck and won't release until you turn off the burner. This can cause some parts of your dish to be overcooked, which can ruin everything you worked so hard to perfect!

Use recipes right away

A great way to use your slow cooker is by developing some new recipes! Have fun experimenting and working on some new ones all at once without having to worry about any nasty flavors ruining your dish later on. Take note of what works well and what does not, so you end up with something delicious every time!

Slow Cookers are a great way to prepare your food and make it taste like someone else has done it for you. With the right recipe in your slow cooker, you can turn days of cooking into hours of preparation.

We've decided to share with you some of our favorite slow cooker recipes from around the country. Some recipes are classic favorites, while others are new and fresh. Whatever you're looking for, you'll find it here.

Slow cookers are a great way to prepare all kinds of meals. With the right recipe, you can cook a variety of dishes, including soups that will warm you up on a cold day.

Some of the advantages to using a slow cooker include reducing the amount of energy needed to use your electric stove. You also don't have to worry about burning yourself when using the stove. You can also leave the slow cooker on when you're not home, making it easy to prepare simple meals and snacks for your family.

You can find many recipes in our slow cooker cookbook. It's divided into several sections, including breakfast, main dishes, side dishes, desserts, and drinks. The slow cooker cookbook is designed for a number of different uses. For example, you can use it to make lots of different side dishes and desserts while you're on vacation or traveling. You can also use the same cookbook in your kitchen to prepare healthy main meals during the week or when you're having friends over for dinner.

Don't let your slow cooker get rusty with age! Contact us today to order our slow cooker cookbook at our guaranteed lowest price. We'll even ship it right away so that you can get started cooking immediately!

Rabbit & Mushroom Stew

Preparation time: 15 minutes

Cooking time: 6 hours

Servings: 6

Ingredients:

- 1 rabbit, in portion size pieces
- 2 cups spicy Spanish sausage, cut into chunks
- 2 Tablespoons butter, divided
- 1 red onion, sliced
- 1 cup button mushrooms, washed and dried
- 1 teaspoon cayenne pepper
- 1 teaspoon sweet paprika
- 1 teaspoon salt
- 1 teaspoon fresh ground black pepper
- 1 cup chicken broth+1 cup hot water

Directions:

1. Butter the slow cooker.
2. In a large pan, melt the butter, add the rabbit pieces, brown on all sides. Transfer to a slow cooker.
3. In the same pan, sauté the onions, sausage chunks, and spices for 2-3 minutes. Set the chicken broth, heat on high for 1 minute, then pour the mixture over the rabbit.
4. Add the mushrooms. Adjust the seasoning, if needed.

5 Add the water. Cover, cook on high for 6 hours. Serve.

Nutrition:

Calories: 122

Carbs: 19g

Fat: 1g

Protein: 10g

Italian Spicy Sausage & Bell Peppers

Preparation time: 15 minutes

Cooking time: 6 hours

Servings: 5

Ingredients:

- 2 Tablespoons butter
- 2 red onions, sliced
- bell peppers, sliced
- 2 regular cans Italian tomatoes, diced
  - pounds spicy Italian sausage
- 1 teaspoon dry oregano
- 1 teaspoon dry thyme
- 1 teaspoon dry basil
- 1 teaspoon sweet paprika
- 1 teaspoon salt
- 1 teaspoon fresh ground black pepper

Directions:

1. Grease with butter the slow cooker. Add the sliced onions and peppers. Salt.
2. Pour the tomatoes over it, then add seasoning. Mix it in.
3. Arrange sausages in the middle of the pepper and onion mixture.
4. Add ¼ cup hot water. Cover, cook on low for 6 hours. Serve.

Nutrition:

Calories: 180

Carbs: 19g

Fat: 6g

Protein: 12g

Chicken in Salsa Verde

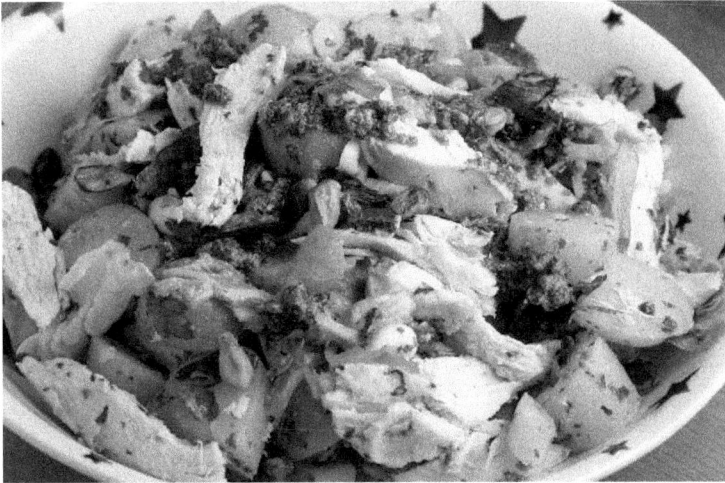

Preparation time: 15 minutes

Cooking time: 6 hours

Servings: 4

Ingredients:

- pounds of chicken breasts
- bunches parsley, chopped
- ¾ cup olive oil
- ¼ cup capers, drained and chopped
- anchovy fillets
- 1 lemon, juice, and zest
- 2 garlic cloves, minced
- 1 teaspoon salt
- 1 teaspoon fresh ground black pepper

Directions:

1. Place the chicken breasts in the slow cooker.
2. Blend the rest of the fixing in a blender, then pour over the chicken.
3. Cover, cook on low for 6 hours. Shred with a fork and serve.

Nutrition:

Calories: 145

Carbs: 5g

Fat: 2g

Protein: 26g

Salmon Poached in White Wine and Lemon

Preparation time: 15 minutes

Cooking time: 2 hours

Servings: 4

Ingredients:

- 2 cups of water
- 1 cup cooking wine, white
- 1 lemon, sliced thin
- 1 small mild onion, sliced thin
- 1 bay leaf
- 1 mixed bunch fresh tarragon, dill, and parsley
  - pounds salmon fillet, skin on
- 1 teaspoon salt
- 1 teaspoon ground black pepper

Directions:

1. Add all fixings, except salmon and seasoning, to the slow cooker. Cover, cook on low for 1 hour.
2. Season the salmon, place in the slow cooker skin-side down.
3. Cover, cook on low for another hour. Serve.

Nutrition:

Calories: 216

Carbs: 1g

Fat: 12g

Protein: 23g

Keto Lasagna

Preparation time: 20 minutes

Cooking time: 7 hours

Servings: 6

Ingredients:

- oz. ground beef

- 1 tablespoon tomato puree

- 1 zucchini

- oz. Parmesan, grated

- 1 tablespoon butter

- ½ teaspoon salt

- 1 teaspoon paprika

- 1 teaspoon chili flakes

- 1 tablespoon full-fat heavy cream

Directions

1   Slice the zucchini lengthwise.

2   Mix the ground beef, salt, paprika, and chili flakes.

3   Then mix the full-fat cream and tomato puree.

4   Chop the butter and put it in the slow cooker.

5   Make a layer of the zucchini in the bottom of the slow cooker bowl.

6   Put a layer of the ground beef mixture on top of the zucchini layer.

7   After this repeat, the same layers until you use all the Ingredients.

8   Sprinkle the lasagna with the grated Parmesan and close the lid.

9   Cook the lasagna for 7 hours on Low.

10   Chill the cooked meal and serve!

Nutrition:

Calories 197,

Fat 11,

Fiber 0.5,

Carbs 2.5, protein 22.5

Butter Chicken

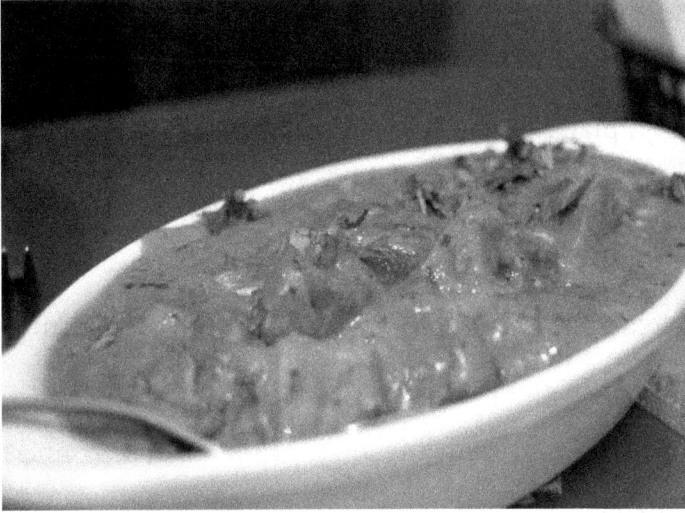

Preparation time: 15 minutes

Cooking time: 3 hours

Servings: 4

Ingredients:

- 1 tablespoons butter

- oz. spinach, chopped

- 1 teaspoon onion powder

- 1 teaspoon paprika

- oz. chicken breast, skinless, boneless

- ½ teaspoon salt

- ¼ cup chicken stock

Directions:

1   Beat the chicken breasts gently to tenderize and sprinkle it with the salt and paprika.

2   Then place the butter and spinach in a blender.

3   Add onion powder and blend the mixture for 1 minute at high speed.

4   Spread the chicken breast with the butter mixture on each side.

5   Place the buttered chicken in the slow cooker and the chicken stock.

6   Close the lid and cook the chicken for 3 hours on Low.

7   Serve the chicken immediately!

Nutrition:

Calories 208,

Fat 13.9,

Fiber 0.7,

Carbs 1.6,

Protein 18.9

Tuscan Chicken

Preparation time: 15 minutes

Cooking time: 7 hours

Servings: 8

Ingredients:

- 1-pound chicken breast, skinless, boneless

- 1 tablespoon olive oil

- ½ cup full-fat cream

- 1 oz. spinach, chopped

- oz. Parmesan, grated

- 1 teaspoon chili flakes

- ½ teaspoon paprika

- 1 teaspoon minced garlic

- ½ teaspoon ground black pepper

Directions:

1   Chop the chicken breast roughly and sprinkle it with the chili flakes, paprika, minced garlic, and ground black pepper.

2   Stir the chicken and transfer to the slow cooker.

3   Add the full-fat cream and olive oil.

4   Add spinach and grated cheese.

5   Stir the chicken gently and close the lid.

6   Cook the chicken for 7 hours on Low.

7   Transfer cooked Tuscan chicken on the serving plates
and serve!

Nutrition:

Calories 136,

Fat 7.2,

Fiber 0.2,

Carbs 1.4, protein 16

Corned Beef

Preparation time: 10 minutes

Cooking time: 8 hours

Servings: 6

Ingredients:

- 1-pound corned beef

- 1 teaspoon peppercorns

- 1 teaspoon chili flakes

- 1 teaspoon mustard seeds

- 1 bay leaf

- 1 teaspoon salt

- 1 oz. bacon fat

- garlic cloves

- 1 cup water

- 1 tablespoon butter

Directions:

1   Mix the peppercorns, chili flakes, mustard seeds, and salt in the bowl.

2   Then rub the corned beef with the spice mixture well.

3   Peel the garlic and place it in the slow cooker.

4   Add the corned beef.

5   Add water, butter, and bay leaf.

6   Add the bacon fat and close the lid.

7   Cook the corned beef for 8 hours on Low.

8   When the corned beef is cooked, discard the bay leaf, then transfer the beef to a plate and cut into servings.

9   Enjoy!

Nutrition:

Calories 178,

Fat 13.5,

Fiber 0.3,

Carbs 1.3,

Protein 12.2

Sardine Pate

Preparation time: 15 minutes

Cooking time: 3 hours

Servings: 6

Ingredients:

- ½ cup water

- 1 tablespoons butter

- 1 teaspoon onion powder

- 1 teaspoon dried parsley

- oz. sardine fillets, chopped

Directions:

1   Put the chopped sardine fillets, dried parsley, onion powder, and water in the slow cooker.

2   Close the lid and cook the fish for 3 hours on Low.

3   Strain the sardine fillet and put it in a blender.

4   Add butter and blend the mixture for 3 minutes at high speed.

5   Transfer the cooked pate into serving bowls and serve!

Nutrition:

Calories 170,

Fat 12.3,

Fiber 0, carbs 0.3,

Protein 14.1

Spare Ribs

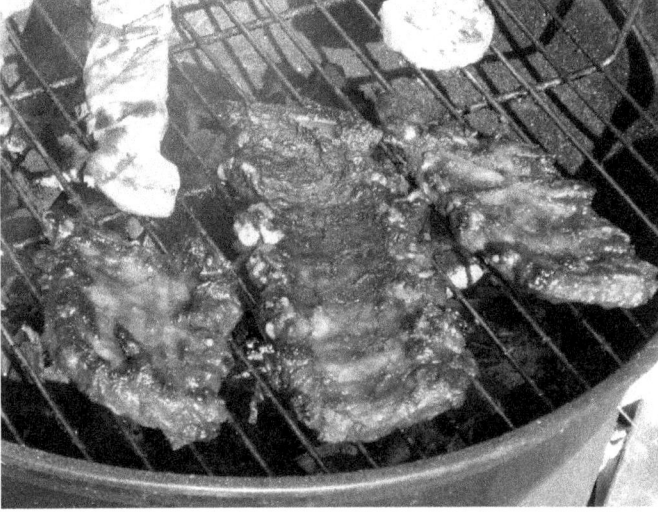

Preparation time: 10 minutes

Cooking time: 8 hours

Servings: 6

Ingredients:

- 1-pound pork loin ribs

- 1 teaspoon olive oil

- 1 teaspoon minced garlic

- ¼ teaspoon cumin

- ¼ teaspoon chili powder

- 1 tablespoon butter

- 1 tablespoons water

Directions:

1   Mix the olive oil, minced garlic, cumin, and chili flakes in a bowl.

2   Melt the butter and add to the spice mixture.

3   Stir it well and add water. Stir again.

4   Then rub the pork ribs with the spice mixture generously and place the ribs in the slow cooker.

5   Close the lid and cook the ribs for 8 hours on Low.

6   When the ribs are cooked, serve them immediately!

Nutrition:

Calories 203,

Fat 14.1, fiber 0.6,

Carbs 10,

Protein 9.8

Pork Shoulder

Preparation time: 25 minutes

Cooking time: 7 hours

Servings: 6

Ingredients:

- 1-pound pork shoulder

- 2 cups water

- 1 onion, peeled

- 2 garlic cloves, peeled

- 1 teaspoon peppercorns

- 1 teaspoon chili flakes

- ½ teaspoon paprika

- 1 teaspoon turmeric

- 1 teaspoon cumin

Directions:

1   Sprinkle the pork shoulder with the peppercorns, chili flakes, paprika, turmeric, and cumin.

2   Stir it well and let it sit for 15 minutes to marinate.

3   Transfer the pork shoulder to the slow cooker.

4   Add water and peeled the onion.

5   Add garlic cloves and close the lid.

6   Cook the pork shoulder for 7 hours on Low.

7   Remove the pork shoulder from the slow cooker and serve!

Nutrition:

Calories 234,

Fat 16.4,

Fiber 0.7,

Carbs 2.8,

Protein 18

Lamb Chops

Preparation time: 15 minutes

Cooking time: 3 hours

Servings: 2

Ingredients:

- oz. lamb chops

- 1 tablespoon tomato puree

- ½ teaspoon cumin

- ½ teaspoon ground coriander

- 1 teaspoon garlic powder

- 1 teaspoon butter

- tablespoons water

Directions:

1   Mix the tomato puree, cumin, ground coriander, garlic powder, and water in the bowl.

2   Brush the lamb chops with the tomato puree mixture on each side and let marinate for 20 minutes.

3   Toss the butter in the slow cooker.

4   Add the lamb chops and close the lid.

5   Cook the lamb chops for 3 hours on High.

6   Transfer the cooked lamb onto serving plates and enjoy!

Nutrition:

Calories 290,

Fat 12.5,

Fiber 0.4,

Carbs 2,

Protein 40.3

Rosemary Leg of Lamb

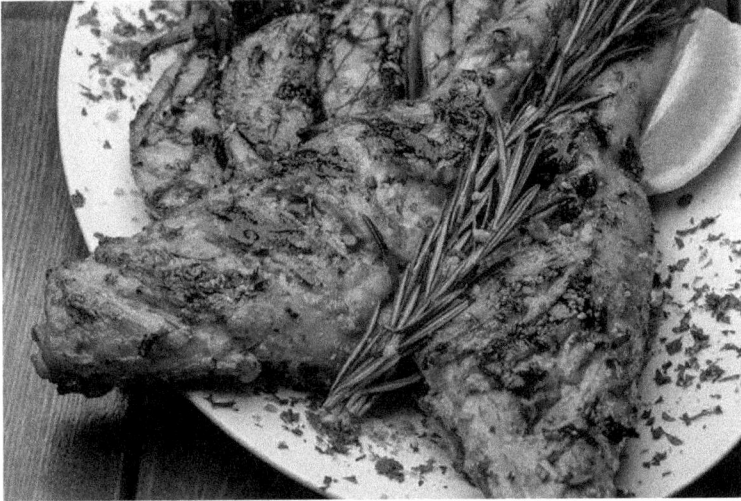

Preparation time: 15 minutes

Cooking time: 7 hours

Servings: 8

Ingredients:

- 2-pound leg of lamb

- 1 onion

- 2 cups water

- 1 garlic clove, peeled

- 1 tablespoon mustard seeds

- 1 teaspoon salt

- ½ teaspoon turmeric
- 1 teaspoon ground black pepper

Directions:

1	Chop the garlic clove and combine it with the mustard seeds, turmeric, black pepper, and salt.

2	Peel the onion and grate it.

3	Mix the grated onion and spice mixture.

4	Rub the leg of lamb with the grated onion mixture.

5	Put the leg of lamb in the slow cooker and cook it for 7 hours on Low.

6	Serve the cooked meal!

Nutrition:

Calories 225,

Fat 8.7,

Fiber 0.6,

Carbs 2.2,

Protein 32.4

Creamy Chicken Thighs

Preparation time: 15 minutes

Cooking time: 6 hours

Servings: 4

Ingredients:

- 1-pound chicken thighs, skinless

- ¼ cup almond milk, unsweetened

- 1 tablespoon full-fat cream cheese

- 1 teaspoon salt

- 1 onion, diced

- 1 teaspoon paprika

Directions

1   Mix the almond milk and full-fat cream.

2   Add salt, diced onion, and paprika.

3   Stir the mixture well.

4   Place the chicken thighs in the slow cooker.

5   Add the almond milk mixture and stir it gently.

6   Close the slow cooker lid and cook the chicken thighs for 6 hours on High.

7   Transfer the cooked chicken thighs into the serving bowls and serve immediately!

Nutrition:

Calories 224,

Fat 14.3,

Fiber 1.1,

Carbs 4.7,

Protein 18.9

Peppered Steak

Preparation time: 15 minutes

Cooking time: 4 hours

Servings: 4

Ingredients:

- oz. Sirloin Steak

- 2 cups water

- 1 tablespoon peppercorns

- 1 teaspoon salt

- ½ teaspoon ground nutmeg

- 2 garlic cloves, peeled

- 1 teaspoon olive oil

Directions:

1   Make the small cuts in the sirloin and chop the garlic cloves roughly.

2   Place the garlic cloves in the sirloin cuts.

3   Sprinkle the steak with the salt, ground nutmeg, and peppercorns.

4   Transfer the steak to the slow cooker and add water.

5   Close the lid and cook the steak for 4 hours on Low.

6   Then remove the steak from the slow cooker and slice it.

7   Enjoy!

Nutrition:

Calories 192,

Fat 12,

Fiber 4,

Carbs 1,

Protein 12

Rabbit Stew

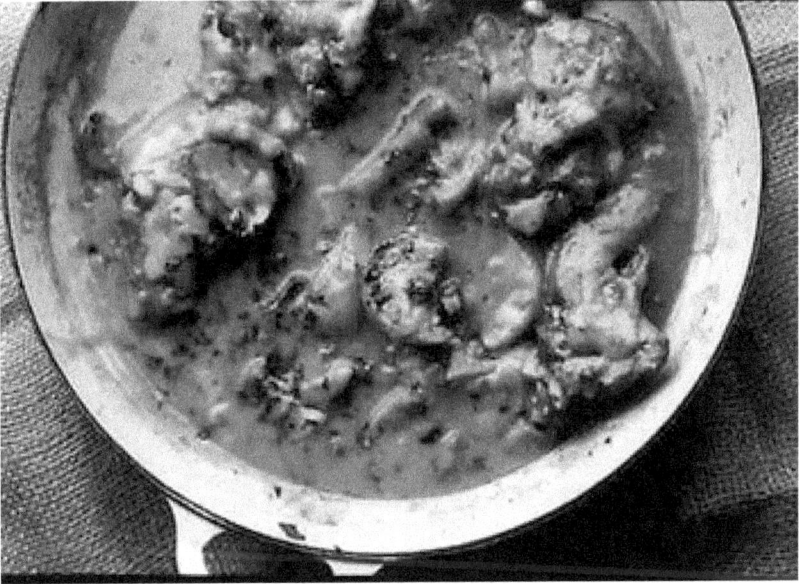

Preparation time: 15 minutes

Cooking time: 5 hours

Servings: 6

Ingredients:

- 2 eggplants, chopped

- 1 zucchini, chopped

- 1 onion, chopped

- oz. rabbit, chopped

- 2 cups water

- 1 tablespoon butter

- 1 teaspoon salt

- 1 teaspoon chili flakes

Directions:

1   Place the chopped eggplants, zucchini, onion, and rabbit in the slow cooker.

2   Add water, butter, salt, and chili flakes.

3   Stir the stew gently and close the lid.

4   Cook the stew for 5 hours on Low.

5   Then let the cooked rabbit stew cool slightly, then serve it!

Nutrition:

Calories 168,

Fat 6.1,

Fiber 7.2,

Carbs 13.6,

Protein 16.1

Duck Breast

Preparation time: 10 minutes

Cooking time: 5 hours

Servings: 4

Ingredients:

- 1 teaspoon liquid stevia

- 1-pound duck breast, boneless, skinless

- 1 teaspoon chili pepper

- 2 tablespoons butter

- ½ cup water

- 1 bay leaf

Directions:

1   Rub the duck breast with the chili pepper and liquid stevia, then transfer it to the slow cooker.

2   Add the bay leaf and water.

3   Add butter and close the lid.

4   Cook the duck breast for 5 hours on Low.

5   Let the cooked duck breast rest for 10 minutes, then remove it from the slow cooker.

6   Slice it into the servings.

7   Enjoy!

Nutrition:

Calories 199

Fat 10.3,

Fiber 0.1,

Carbs 0.3,

Protein 25.1

Jerk Chicken

Preparation time: 25 minutes

Cooking time: 5 hours

Servings: 4

Ingredients:

- 1 teaspoon nutmeg

- 1 teaspoon cinnamon

- 1 teaspoon minced garlic

- ½ teaspoon cloves

- 1 teaspoon ground coriander

- 1 tablespoon Erythritol

- 1-pound chicken thighs

- ½ cup water

- 1 tablespoon butter

Directions:

1   Mix the nutmeg, cinnamon, minced garlic, cloves, and ground coriander.

2   Add Erythritol and stir the **Ingredients:** until well blended.

3   Sprinkle the chicken thighs with the spice mixture.

4   Let the chicken thighs sit for 10 minutes to marinate, then put the chicken thighs in the slow cooker.

5   Add the butter and water.

6   Close the lid and cook Jerk chicken for 5 hours on Low.

7   Serve Jerk chicken immediately!

Nutrition:

Calories 247,

Fat 11.5,

Fiber 0.5,

Carbs 4.9,

Protein 33

Balsamic Beef

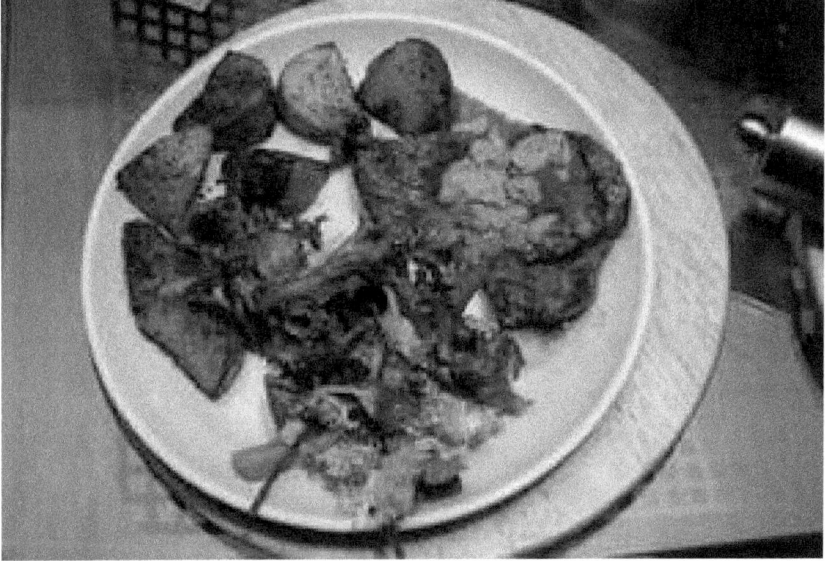

Preparation time: 20 minutes

Cooking time: 7 hours

Servings: 4

Ingredients:

- 2 tablespoons balsamic vinegar

- 1 tablespoon olive oil

- 1-pound beef loin

- 1 teaspoon minced garlic

- ½ teaspoon ground coriander

- 1 teaspoon cumin

- ½ teaspoon dried dill

- 2 tablespoons water

Directions:

1   Chop the beef loin roughly and place it in a large bowl, then sprinkle it with the balsamic vinegar.

2   Add olive oil, minced garlic, ground coriander, cumin, and dried dill.

3   Stir the meat well and let sit for 10 minutes.

4   Place the meat in the slow cooker and add water.

5   Close the lid and cook the beef for 7 hours on Low.

6   When the beef is tender, it is cooked!

7   Enjoy!

Nutrition:

Calories 241,

Fat 13.1,

Fiber 0.1,

Carbs 0.6,

Protein 30.5

Onion Beef

Preparation time: 10 minutes

Cooking time: 5.5 hours

Servings: 14

Ingredients:

- 4-pounds beef sirloin, sliced

- 2 cups white onion, chopped

- 2 cups of water

- ½ cup butter

- 1 teaspoon ground black pepper

- 1 teaspoon salt

- 1 bay leaf

Directions

1   Mix beef sirloin with salt and ground black pepper and transfer to the slow cooker.

2   Add butter, water, onion, and bay leaf.

3   Close the lid and cook the meat on High for 5.5 hours.

Nutrition :

306 calories,

39.6g protein,

1.7g carbohydrates,

14.7g fat,

0.4g fiber,

133mg cholesterol,

301mg sodium,

551mg potassium.

Cilantro Beef

Preparation time: 10 minutes

Cooking time: 4.5 hours

Servings: 4

Ingredients:

- 1-pound beef loin, roughly chopped

- ¼ cup apple cider vinegar

- 1 tablespoon dried cilantro

- ½ teaspoon dried basil

- 1 cup of water

- 1 teaspoon tomato paste

Direction

1   Mix meat with tomato paste, dried cilantro, and basil.

2   Then transfer it to the slow cooker.

3   Add apple cider vinegar and water.

4   Cook the cilantro beef for 4.5 hours on High.

Nutrition

211 calories,

30.4g protein,

0.4g carbohydrates,

9.5g fat,

0.1g fiber,

81mg cholesterol,

66mg sodium,

412mg potassium.

Garlic Sweet Potato

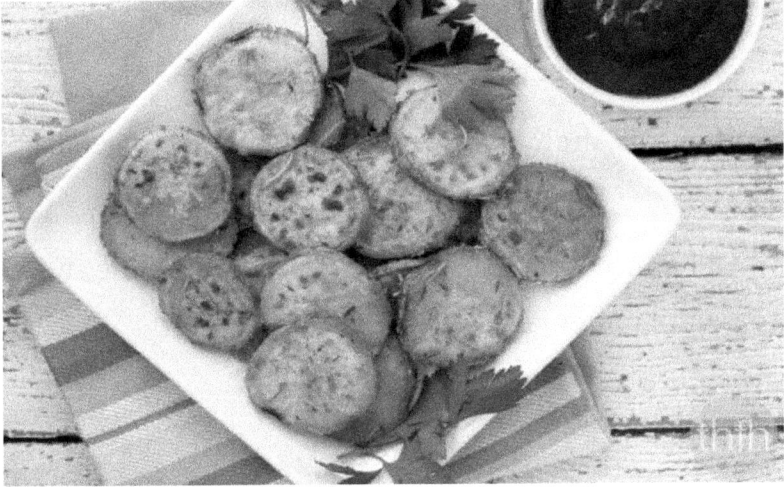

Preparation time: 10 minutes

Cooking time: 6 hours

Servings: 4

Ingredients:

- 2-pounds sweet potatoes, chopped

- 1 teaspoon minced garlic

- tablespoons vegan butter

- 1 teaspoon salt

- water

Directions

1   Pour water into the slow cooker. Add sweet potatoes.

2   Then add salt and close the lid.

3   Cook the sweet potato on Low for 6 hours.

4   After this, drain the water and transfer the vegetables in the big bowl.

5   Add minced garlic and butter. Carefully stir the sweet potatoes until butter is melted.

Nutrition

320 calories,

3.6g protein,

63.5g carbohydrates,

6.2g fat,

9.3g fiber,

15mg cholesterol,

648mg sodium,

1857mg potassium.

Potato Salad

Preparation time: 10 minutes

Cooking time: 3 hours

Servings: 2

Ingredients:

- 1 cup potato, chopped

- 1 cup of water

- 1 teaspoon salt

- oz. celery stalk, chopped

- oz. fresh parsley, chopped

- ¼ onion, diced

- 1 tablespoon mayonnaise

Directions

1   Put the potatoes in the slow cooker.

2   Add water and salt.

3   Cook the potatoes on High for 3 hours.

4   Then drain water and transfer the potatoes in the salad bowl.

5   Add all remaining **Ingredients:** and carefully mix the salad.

Nutrition

129 calories,

5.5g protein,

12.4g carbohydrates,

6.7g fat,

2.5g fiber,

12mg cholesterol,

1479mg sodium,

465mg potassium.

Sautéed Greens

Preparation time: 15 minutes

Cooking time: 1 hour

Servings: 4

Ingredients:

- 1 cup spinach, chopped

- 2 cups collard greens, chopped

- 1 cup Swiss chard, chopped

- water

- ½ cup half and half

Directions

1 Put spinach, collard greens, and Swiss chard in the slow cooker.

2 Add water and close the lid.

3 Cook the greens on High for 1 hour.

4 Then drain water and transfer the greens in the bowl.

5 Bring the half and half to boil and pour over greens.

6 Carefully mix the greens.

Nutrition

49 calories,

1.8g protein,

3.2g carbohydrates,

3.7g fat,

1.1g fiber,

11mg cholesterol,

45mg sodium,

117mg potassium.

Mashed Turnips

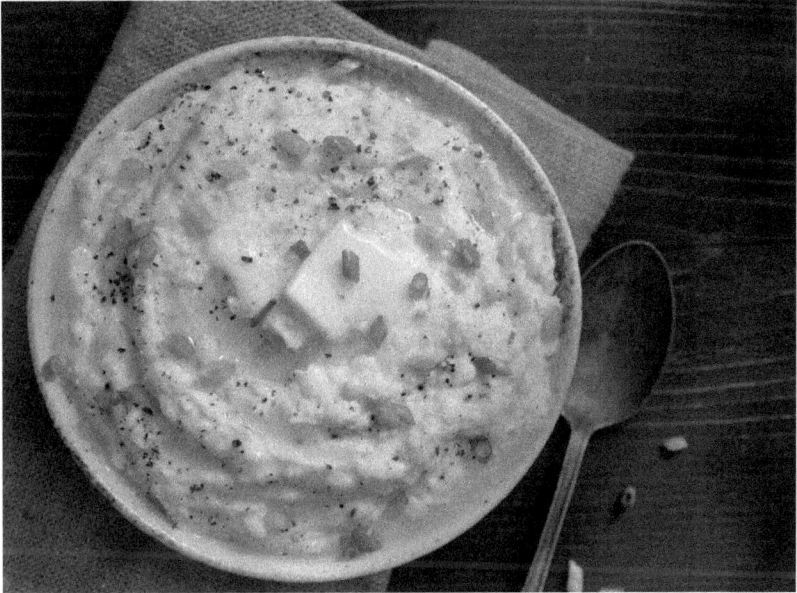

Preparation time: 10 minutes

Cooking time: 7 hours

Servings: 6

Ingredients:

- 3-pounds turnip, chopped

- 2 cup water

- 1 tablespoon vegan butter

- 1 tablespoon chives, chopped

- oz. Parmesan, grated

Directions

1   Put turnips in the slow cooker.

2   Add water and cook the vegetables on low for 7 hours.

3   Then drain water and mash the turnips.

4   Add chives, butter, and Parmesan.

5   Carefully stir the mixture until butter and Parmesan are melted.

6   Then add chives. Mix the mashed turnips again.

Nutrition

162 calories,

8.6g protein,

15.1g carbohydrates,

8.1g fat,

4.1g fiber,

22mg cholesterol,

475mg sodium,

490mg potassium.

Cilantro Meatballs

Preparation time: 20 minutes

Cooking time: 4 hours

Servings: 6

Ingredients:

- 1-pound minced beef

- 1 teaspoon minced garlic

- 1 egg, beaten

- 1 teaspoon chili flakes

- 2 teaspoons dried cilantro

- 1 tablespoon semolina

- ½ cup of water

- 1 tablespoon sesame oil

Directions

1   In the bowl, mix minced beef, garlic, egg, chili flakes, cilantro, and semolina.

2   Then make the meatballs.

3   After this, heat the sesame oil in the skillet.

4   Cook the meatballs in the hot oil on high heat for 1 minute per side.

5   Transfer the roasted meatballs to the slow cooker, add water, and close the lid.

6   Cook the meatballs on High for 4 hours.

Nutrition :

178 calories,

24.1g protein,

1.5g carbohydrates,

7.7g fat,

0.1g fiber,

95mg cholesterol,

61mg sodium,

321mg potassium.

Stuffed Jalapenos

Preparation time: 10 minutes

Cooking time: 4.5 hours

Servings: 3

Ingredients:

- jalapenos, deseed

- oz. minced beef

- 1 teaspoon garlic powder

- ½ cup of water

Directions

1   Mix the minced beef with garlic powder.

2   Then fill the jalapenos with minced meat and arrange it in the slow cooker.

3   Add water and cook the jalapenos on High for 4.5 hours.

Nutrition :

55 calories,

7.5g protein,

2.3g carbohydrates,

1.9g fat,

0.9g fiber,

0mg cholesterol,

2mg sodium,

71mg potassium.

BBQ Beef Short Ribs

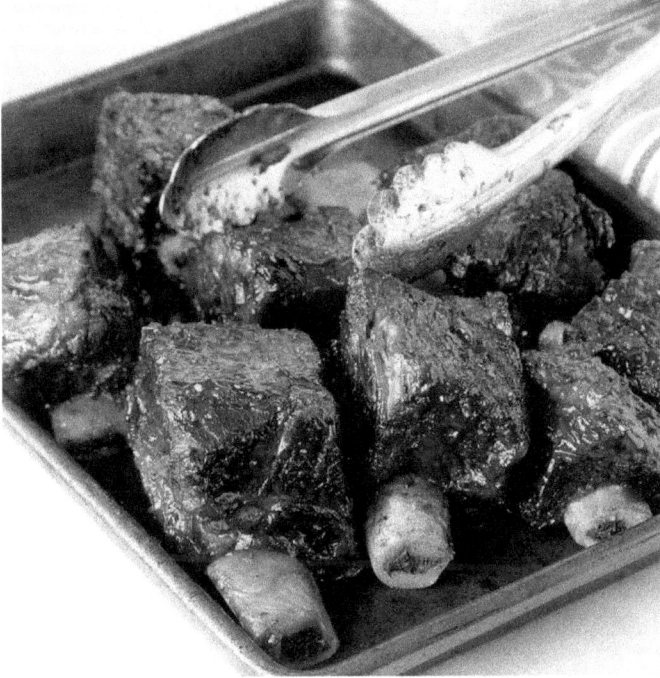

Preparation time: 10 minutes

Cooking time: 5 hours

Servings: 4

Ingredients:

- 1-pound beef short ribs

- ¼ cup of water

- 1/3 cup BBQ sauce

- 1 teaspoon chili powder

Directions

1	Rub the beef short ribs with chili powder and put in the slow cooker.

2	Mix water with BBQ sauce and pour the liquid into the slow cooker.

3	Cook the meat on High for 5 hours.

Nutrition :

266 calories,

32.8g protein,

7.9g carbohydrates,

10.4g fat,

0.3g fiber,

103mg cholesterol,

308mg sodium,

468mg potassium.

Spiced Beef

Preparation time: 10 minutes

Cooking time: 9 hours

Servings: 4

Ingredients:

- 1-pound beef loin

- 1 teaspoon allspice

- 1 teaspoon olive oil

- 1 tablespoon minced onion

- 1 cup of water

Directions

1   Rub the beef loin with allspice, olive oil, and minced onion.

2   Put the meat in the slow cooker.

3   Add water and close the lid.

4   Cook the beef on Low for 9 hours.

5   When the meat is cooked, slice it into servings.

Nutrition:

219 calories,

30.4g protein,

0.6g carbohydrates,

10.7g fat,

0.2g fiber,

81mg cholesterol,

65mg sodium,

395mg potassium.

Green Peas Chowder

Preparation time: 10 minutes

Cooking time: 8 hours

Servings: 6

Ingredients:

- 1-pound chicken breast, skinless, boneless, chopped

- 2 cups water

- 1 cup green peas

- ¼ cup Greek Yogurt

- 1 tablespoon dried basil

- 1 teaspoon ground black pepper

- ½ teaspoon salt

Directions

1   Mix salt, chicken breast, ground black pepper, and dried basil.

2   Transfer the **Ingredients:** to the slow cooker.

3   Add water, green peas, yogurt, and close the lid.

4   Cook the chowder on Low for 8 hours.

Nutrition:

113 calories,

18.2g protein,

4.1g carbohydrates,

2.2g fat,

1.3g fiber,

49mg cholesterol,

244mg sodium,

359mg potassium.

Chorizo Soup

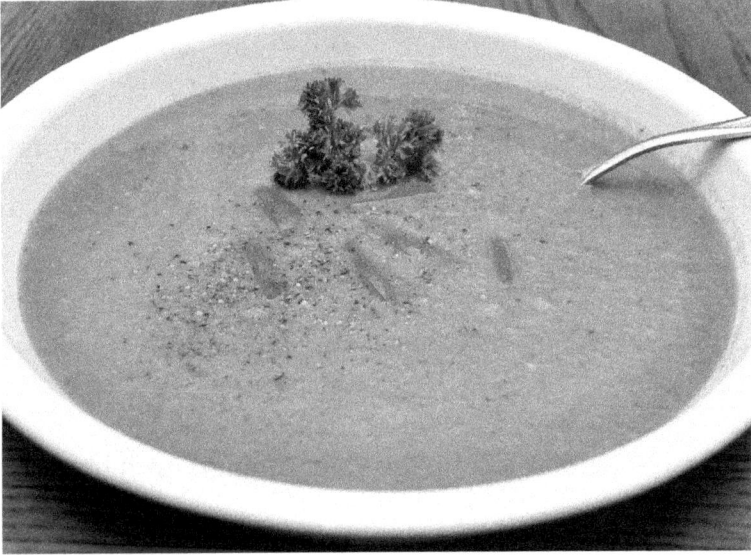

Preparation time: 10 minutes

Cooking time: 5 hours

Servings: 6

Ingredients:

- oz. chorizo, chopped

- 2 cup water

- 1 cup potato, chopped

- 1 teaspoon minced garlic, chopped

- 1 zucchini, chopped

- ½ cup spinach, chopped

- 1 teaspoon salt

Directions

1   Put the chorizo in the skillet and roast it for 2 minutes per side on high heat.

2   Then transfer the chorizo to the slow cooker.

3   Add water, potato, minced garlic, zucchini, spinach, and salt.

4   Close the lid and cook the soup on high for 5 hours.

5   Then cool the soup to room temperature.

Nutrition :

210 calories,

11g protein,

4.3g carbohydrates,

16.4g fat,

0.7g fiber,

37mg cholesterol,

927mg sodium,

326mg potassium.

Aromatic Jalapeno Wings

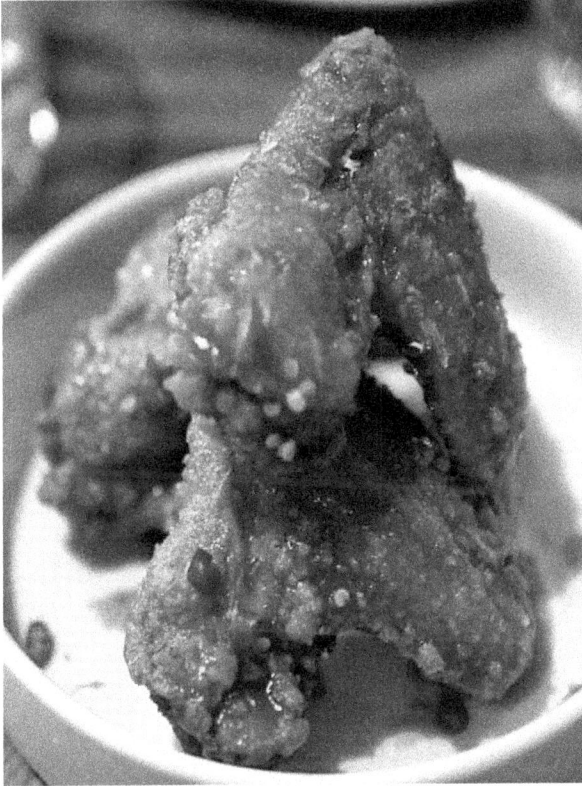

Preparation time: 10 minutes

Cooking time: 3 hours

Servings: 4

Ingredients:

- 1 jalapeño pepper, diced

- ½ cup of fresh cilantro, diced

- 3 tablespoon of coconut oil

- Juice from 1 lime

- 2 garlic cloves, peeled and minced

- Salt and black pepper ground, to taste

- 2 lbs. chicken wings

- Lime wedges, to serve

- Mayonnaise, to serve

Directions:

1. Start by throwing all the Ingredients into the large bowl and mix well.

2. Cover the wings and marinate them in the refrigerator for 2 hours.

3. Now add the wings along with their marinade into the Slow cooker.

4. Cover it and cook for 3 hours on Low Settings.

5. Garnish as desired.

6. Serve warm.

Nutrition:

Calories 246

Total Fat 7.4 g

Saturated Fat 4.6 g

Cholesterol 105 mg

Total Carbs 9.4 g

Sugar 6.5 g

Fiber 2.7 g

Sodium 353 mg

Potassium 529 mg

Protein 37.2 g

Barbeque Chicken Wings

Preparation time: 10 minutes

Cooking time: 3 hours

Servings: 4

Ingredients:

- 2 lbs. chicken wings
- 1/2 cup of water
- 1/2 teaspoon of basil, dried
- 3/4 cup of BBQ sauce
- 1/2 cup of lime juice
- 1 teaspoon of red pepper, crushed
- 2 teaspoons of paprika
- 1/2 cup of swerve
- Salt and black pepper- to taste
- A pinch cayenne peppers

Directions:

1. Start by throwing all the Ingredients into the Slow cooker and mix them well.
2. Cover it and cook for 3 hours on Low Settings.
3. Garnish as desired.

4. Serve warm.

Nutrition:

Calories 457

Total Fat 19.1 g

Saturated Fat 11 g

Cholesterol 262 mg

Total Carbs 8.9 g

Sugar 1.2 g

Fiber 1.7 g

Sodium 557 mg

Potassium 748 mg

Protein 32.5 g

Saucy Duck

Preparation time: 10 minutes

Cooking time: 6 hours

Servings: 4

Ingredients

- 1 duck, cut into small chunks

- 4 garlic cloves, minced

- 4 tablespoons of swerves

- 2 green onions, roughly diced

- 4 tablespoon of soy sauce

- 4 tablespoon of sherry wine

- 1/4 cup of water

- 1-inch ginger root, sliced

- A pinch salt

- black pepper to taste

Directions:

1. Start by throwing all the Ingredients into the Slow cooker and mix them well.

2. Cover it and cook for 6 hours on Low Settings.

3. Garnish as desired.

4. Serve warm.

Nutrition:

Calories 338

Total Fat 3.8 g

Saturated Fat 0.7 g

Cholesterol 22 mg

Total Carbs 8.3 g

Fiber 2.4 g

Sugar 1.2 g

Sodium 620 mg

Potassium 271 mg

Protein 15.4g

Chicken Roux Gumbo

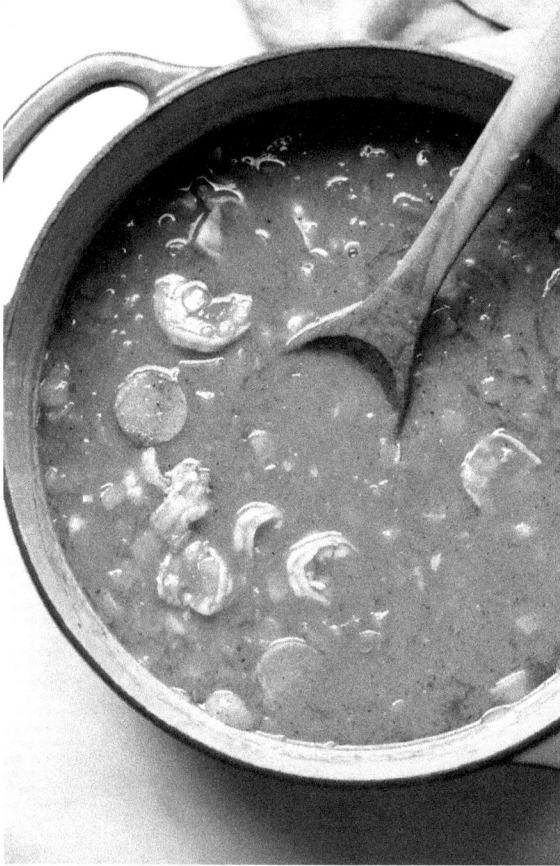

Preparation time: 10 minutes

Cooking time: 6 hours

Servings: 24

Ingredients:

- 1 lb. chicken thighs, cut into halves

- 1 tablespoon of vegetable oil

- 1 lb. smoky sausage, sliced, crispy, and crumbled.

- Salt and black pepper- to taste

Aromatics:

- 1 bell pepper, diced

- 2 quarts' chicken stock

- 15 oz. canned tomatoes, diced

- 1 celery stalk, diced

- salt to taste

- 4 garlic cloves, minced

- 1/2 lbs. okra, sliced

- 1 yellow onion, diced

- a dash tabasco sauce

For the roux:

- 1/2 cup of almond flour

- 1/4 cup of vegetable oil

- 1 teaspoon of Cajun spice

Directions:

1. Start by throwing all the Ingredients except okra and roux Ingredients into the Slow cooker.

2. Cover it and cook for 5 hours on Low Settings.

3. Stir in okra and cook for another 1 hour on low heat.

4. Mix all the roux Ingredients and add them to the Slow cooker.

5. Stir cook on high heat until the sauce thickens.

6. Garnish as desired.

7. Serve warm.

Nutrition:

Calories 604

Total Fat 30.6 g

Saturated Fat 13.1 g

Cholesterol 131 mg

Total Carbs 1.4g

Fiber 0.2 g

Sugar 20.3 g

Sodium 834 mg

Potassium 512 mg

Protein 54.6 g

Cider-Braised Chicken

Preparation time: 10 minutes

Cooking time: 5 hours

Servings: 2

Ingredients:

- 4 chicken drumsticks

- 2 tablespoon of olive oil

- ½ cup of apple cider vinegar

- 1 tablespoon of balsamic vinegar

- 1 chili pepper, diced

- 1 yellow onion, minced

- Salt and black pepper- to taste

Directions:

1. Start by throwing all the Ingredients into a bowl and mix them well.

2. Marinate this chicken for 2 hours in the refrigerator.

3. Spread the chicken along with its marinade in the Slow cooker.

4. Cover it and cook for 5 hours on Low Settings.

5. Garnish as desired.

6. Serve warm.

Nutrition:

- Calories 311

- Total Fat 25.5 g

- Saturated Fat 12.4 g

- Cholesterol 69 mg

- Total Carbs 1.4 g

- Fiber 0.7 g

- Sugar 0.3 g

- Sodium 58 mg

- Potassium 362 mg

- Protein 18.4 g

Chunky Chicken Salsa

Preparation time: 10 minutes

Cooking time: 6 hours

Servings: 2

Ingredients

- 1 lb. chicken breast, skinless and boneless

- 1 cup of chunky salsa

- 3/4 teaspoon of cumin

- A pinch oregano

- Salt and black pepper- to taste

Directions:

1. Start by throwing all the Ingredients into the Slow cooker and mix them well.

2. Cover it and cook for 6 hours on Low Settings.

3. Garnish as desired.

4. Serve warm.

Nutrition:

Calories 541

Total Fat 34 g

Saturated Fat 8.5 g

Cholesterol 69 mg

Total Carbs 3.4 g

Fiber 1.2 g

Sugar 1 g

Sodium 547 mg

Potassium 467 mg

Protein 20.3 g

Dijon Chicken

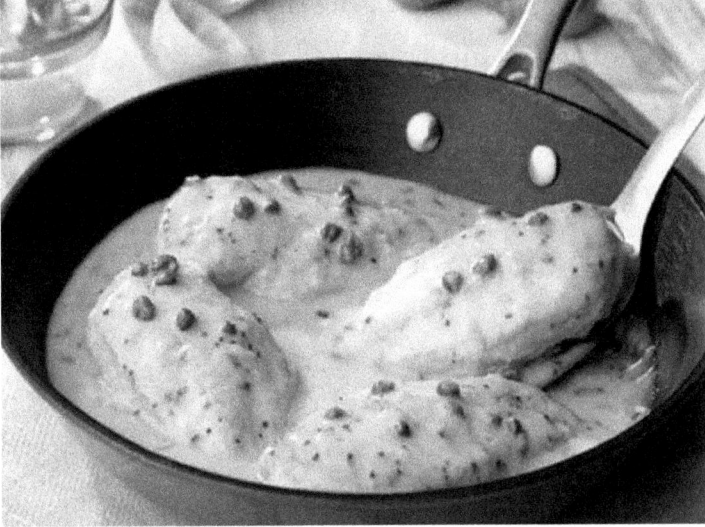

Preparation time: 10 minutes

Cooking time: 6 hours

Servings: 4

Ingredients:

- 2 lbs. chicken thighs, skinless and boneless

- 3/4 cup of chicken stock

- 1/4 cup of lemon juice

- 2 tablespoon of extra virgin olive oil

- 3 tablespoon of Dijon mustard

- 2 tablespoons of Italian seasoning

- Salt and black pepper- to taste

Directions:

1. Start by throwing all the Ingredients into the Slow cooker and mix them well.

2. Cover it and cook for 6 hours on Low Settings.

3. Garnish as desired.

4. Serve warm.

Nutrition:

Calories 398

Total Fat 13.8 g

Saturated Fat 5.1 g

Cholesterol 200 mg

Total Carbs 3.6 g

Fiber 1 g

Sugar 1.3 g

Sodium 272 mg

Potassium 531 mg

Protein 51.8 g

Chicken Thighs with Vegetables

Preparation time: 10 minutes

Cooking time: 6 hours

Servings: 6

Ingredients

- 6 chicken thighs

- 1 teaspoon of vegetable oil

- 15 oz. canned tomatoes, diced

- 1 yellow onion, diced

- 2 tablespoon of tomato paste

- 1/2 cup of white wine

- 2 cups of chicken stock

- 1 celery stalk, diced

- 1/4 lb. baby carrots, cut into halves

- 1/2 teaspoon of thyme, dried

- Salt and black pepper- to taste

Directions:

1. Start by throwing all the Ingredients into the Slow cooker and mix them well.

2. Cover it and cook for 6 hours on Low Settings.

3. Shred the slow-cooked chicken using a fork and return to the pot.

4. Mix well and garnish as desired.

5. Serve warm.

Nutrition:

Calories 372

Total Fat 11.8 g

Saturated Fat 4.4 g

Cholesterol 62 mg

Total Carbs 1.8 g

Fiber 0.6 g

Sugar 27.3 g

Sodium 871 mg

Potassium 288 mg

Protein 34 g

Chicken dipped in tomatillo Sauce

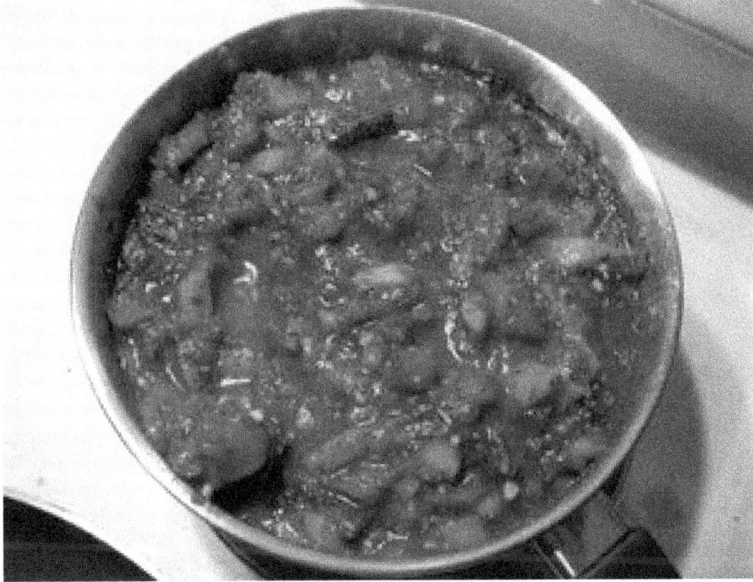

Preparation time: 10 minutes

Cooking time: 6 hours

Servings: 4

Ingredients:

- 1 lb. chicken thighs, skinless and boneless

- 2 tablespoon of extra virgin olive oil

- 1 yellow onion, sliced

- 1 garlic clove, crushed

- 4 oz. canned green chilies, diced

- 1 handful cilantro, diced

- 15 oz. cauliflower rice, already cooked

- 5 oz. tomatoes, diced

- 15 oz. cheddar cheese, grated

- 4 oz. black olives, pitted and diced

- Salt and black pepper- to taste

- 15 oz. canned tomatillos, diced

Directions:

1. Start by throwing all the Ingredients into the Slow cooker and mix them well.

2. Cover it and cook for 5 6 hours on Low Settings.

3. Shred the slow-cooked chicken and return to the pot.

4. Mix well and garnish as desired.

5. Serve warm.

Nutrition:

Calories 427

Total Fat 31.1 g

Saturated Fat 4.2 g

Cholesterol 0 mg

Total Carbs 9 g

Sugar 12.4 g

Fiber 19.8 g

Sodium 86 mg

Potassium 100 mg

Protein 23.5 g

Chicken with Lemon Parsley Butter

Preparation time: 10 minutes

Cooking time: 3 hours

Servings: 10

Ingredients:

- 1 (5 – 6lbs) whole roasting chicken, rinsed

- 1 cup of water

- 1/2 teaspoon of kosher salt

- 1/4 teaspoon of black pepper

- 1 whole lemon, sliced

- 4 tablespoons of butter

- 2 tablespoons of fresh parsley, chopped

Directions:

1. Start by seasoning the chicken with all the herbs and spices.

2. Place this chicken in the Slow cooker.

3. Cover it and cook for 3 hours on High Settings.

4. Meanwhile, melt butter with lemon slices and parsley in a saucepan.

5. Drizzle the butter over the Slow cooker chicken.

6. Serve warm.

Nutrition:

Calories 379

Total Fat 29.7 g

Saturated Fat 18.6 g

Cholesterol 141 mg

Total Carbs 9.7g

Fiber 0.9 g

Sugar 1.3 g

Sodium 193 mg

Potassium 131 mg

Protein 25.2 g

Paprika Chicken

Preparation time: 10 minutes

Cooking time: 8 hours

Servings: 8

Ingredients:

- 1 free-range whole chicken
- 1 tablespoon of olive oil
- 1 tablespoon of dried paprika
- 1 tablespoon of curry powder
- 1 teaspoon of dried turmeric
- 1 teaspoon of salt

Directions:

1. Start by mixing all the spices and oil in a bowl except chicken.
2. Now season the chicken with these spices liberally.
3. Add the chicken and spices to your Slow cooker.
4. Cover the lid of the slow cooker and cook for 8 hours on Low.
5. Serve warm.

Nutrition:

Calories 313

Total Fat 134g

Saturated Fat 78 g

Cholesterol 861 mg

Total Carbs 6.3 g

Fiber 0.7 g

Sugar 19 g

Sodium 62 mg

Potassium 211 mg

Protein 24.6 g

Rotisserie Chicken

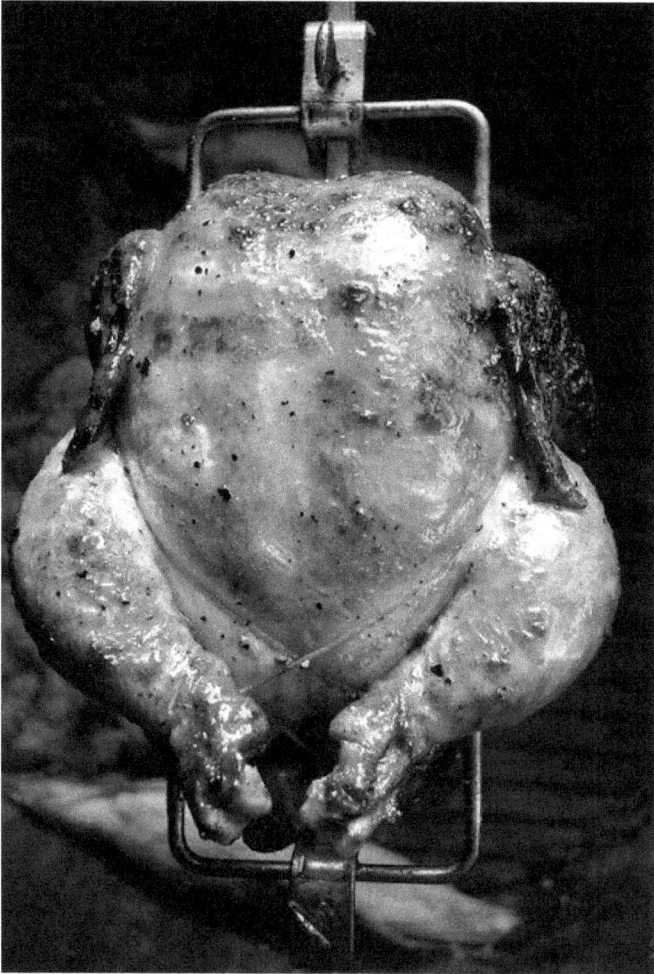

Preparation time: 10 minutes

Cooking time: 8 hours 5 minutes

Servings: 10

Ingredients:

- 1 organic whole chicken

- 1 tablespoon of olive oil

- 1 teaspoon of thyme

- 1 teaspoon of rosemary

- 1 teaspoon of garlic, granulated

- salt and pepper

Directions:

1. Start by seasoning the chicken with all the herbs and spices.

2. Broil this seasoned chicken for 5 minutes in the oven until golden brown.

3. Place this chicken in the Slow cooker.

4. Cover it and cook for 8 hours on Low Settings.

5. Serve warm.

Nutrition:

Calories 301

Total Fat 12.2 g

Saturated Fat 2.4 g

Cholesterol 110 mg

Total Carbs 2.5 g

Fiber 0.9 g

Sugar 1.4 g

Sodium 276 mg

Potassium 231 mg

Protein 28.8 g

Slow cooker Chicken Adobo

Preparation time: 10 minutes

Cooking time: 8 hours

Servings: 6

Ingredients:

- 1/4 cup of apple cider vinegar

- 12 chicken drumsticks

- 1 onion, diced into slices

- 2 tablespoons of olive oil

- 10 cloves garlic, smashed

- 1 cup of gluten-free tamari

- 1/4 cup of diced green onion

Directions:

1. Place the drumsticks in the Slow cooker and then add the remaining Ingredients on top.

2. Cover it and cook for 8 hours on Low Settings.

3. Mix gently, then serve warm.

Nutrition:

Calories 249

Total Fat 11.9 g

Saturated Fat 1.7 g

Cholesterol 78 mg

Total Carbs 1.8 g

Fiber 1.1 g

Sugar 0.3 g

Sodium 79 mg

Potassium 131 mg

Protein 25 g

Chicken Ginger Curry

Preparation time: 10 minutes

Cooking time: 6 hours

Servings: 4

Ingredients:

- 1 ½ lbs. chicken drumsticks (approx. 5 drumsticks), skin removed
- 1 (13.5 oz.) can coconut milk
- 1 onion, diced
- 4 cloves garlic, minced
- 1-inch knob fresh ginger, minced
- 1 Serrano pepper, minced
- 1 tablespoon of Garam Masala
- ½ teaspoon of cayenne
- ½ teaspoon of paprika
- ½ teaspoon of turmeric
- salt and pepper, adjust to taste

Directions:

1. Start by throwing all the Ingredients into the Slow cooker.

2. Cover it and cook for 6 hours on Low Settings.

3. Garnish as desired.

4. Serve warm.

Nutrition:

Calories 248

Total Fat 15.7 g

Saturated Fat 2.7 g

Cholesterol 75 mg

Total Carbs 8.4 g

Fiber 0g

Sugar 1.1 g

Sodium 94 mg

Potassium 331 mg

Protein 14.1 g

Thai Chicken Curry

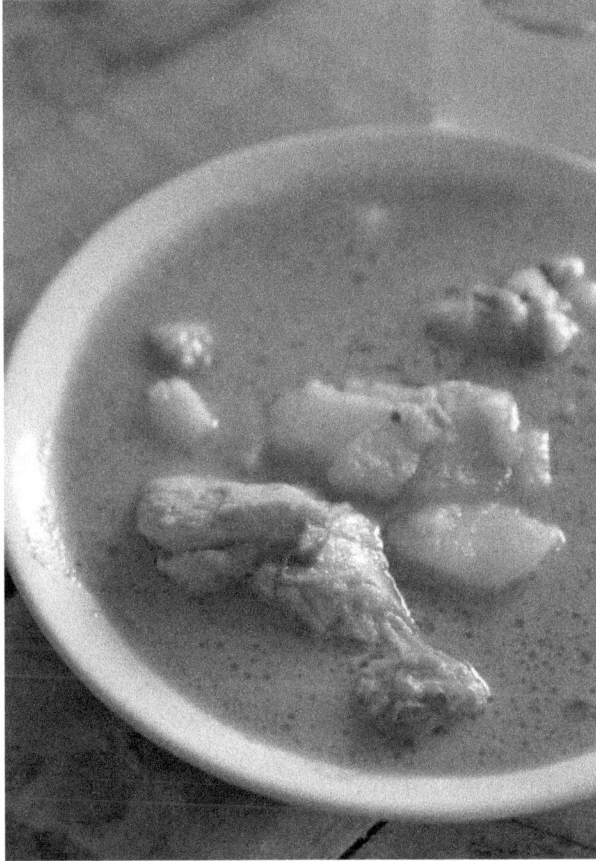

Preparation time: 10 minutes

Cooking time: 2.5 hours

Servings: 2

Ingredients:

- 1 can coconut milk

- 1/2 cup of chicken stock

- 1 lb. boneless, skinless chicken thighs, diced

- 1 2 tablespoons of red curry paste

- 1 tablespoon of coconut aminos

- 1 tablespoon of fish sauce

- 2 3 garlic cloves, minced

- Salt and black pepper-to taste

- red pepper flakes as desired

- 1 bag frozen mixed veggies

Directions:

1. Start by throwing all the Ingredient except vegetables into the Slow cooker.

2. Cover it and cook for 2 hours on Low Settings.

3. Remove its lid and thawed veggies.

4. Cover the slow cooker again then continue cooking for another 30 minutes on Low settings.

5. Garnish as desired.

6. Serve warm.

Nutrition:

Calories 327

Total Fat 3.5 g

Saturated Fat 0.5 g

Cholesterol 162 mg

Total Carbs 56g

Fiber 0.4 g

Sugar 0.5 g

Sodium 142 mg

Potassium 558 mg

Protein 21.5 g

Lemongrass and Coconut Chicken Drumsticks

Preparation time: 10 minutes

Cooking time: 5 hours

Servings: 5

Ingredients:

- 10 drumsticks, skin removed
- 1 thick stalk fresh lemongrass
- 4 cloves garlic, minced
- 1 thumb-size piece of ginger
- 1 cup of coconut milk
- 2 tablespoons of Red Boat fish sauce
- 3 tablespoons of coconut aminos
- 1 teaspoon of five-spice powder
- 1 large onion, sliced
- ¼ cup of fresh scallions, diced
- Kosher salt
- Black pepper

Directions:

1. Start by throwing all the Ingredient into the Slow cooker.

2. Cover it and cook for 5 hours on Low Settings.

3. Garnish as desired.

4. Serve warm.

Nutrition:

Calories 372

Total Fat 11.1 g

Saturated Fat 5.8 g

Cholesterol 610 mg

Total Carbs 0.9 g

Fiber 0.2 g

Sugar 0.2 g

Sodium 749 mg

Potassium 488 mg

Protein 63.5 g

Green Chile Chicken

Preparation time: 10 minutes

Cooking time: 6 hours

Servings: 6

Ingredients:

- 8 chicken thighs, thawed, boneless and skinless

- 1 (4 oz.) can green chilis

- 2 teaspoons of garlic salt

- optional: add in ½ cup of diced onions

Directions:

1. Start by throwing all the Ingredients into the Slow cooker.

2. Cover it and cook for 6 hours on Low Settings.

3. Garnish as desired.

4. Serve warm.

Nutrition:

Calories 248

Total Fat 2.4 g

Saturated Fat 0.1 g

Cholesterol 320 mg

Total Carbs 2.9 g

Fiber 0.7 g

Sugar 0.7 g

Sodium 350 mg

Potassium 255 mg

Protein 44.3 g

Garlic Butter Chicken with Cream Cheese Sauce

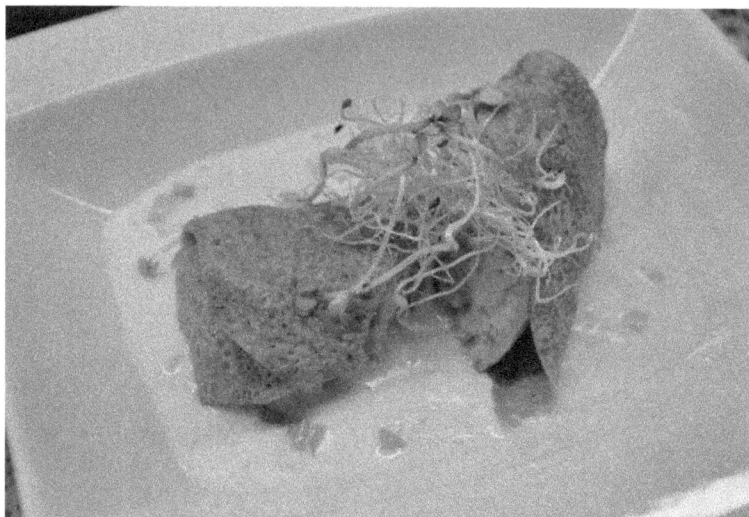

Preparation time: 10 minutes

Cooking time: 6 hours

Servings: 4

Ingredients:

For the garlic chicken:

- 8 garlic cloves, sliced
- 1.5 teaspoons of salt
- 1 stick of butter
- 2 2.5 lbs. of chicken breasts

- Optional 1 onion, sliced

For the cream cheese sauce:

- 8 oz. of cream cheese

- 1 cup of chicken stock

- salt to taste

Directions:

1. Start by throwing all the Ingredients for garlic chicken into the Slow cooker.

2. Cover it and cook for 6 hours on Low Settings.

3. Now stir cook all the Ingredients for cream cheese sauce in a saucepan.

4. Once heated, pour this sauce over the cooked chicken.

5. Garnish as desired.

6. Serve warm.

Nutrition:

- Calories 301

Total Fat 12.2 g

Saturated Fat 2.4 g

Cholesterol 110 mg

Total Carbs 1.5 g

Fiber 0.9 g

Sugar 1.4 g

Sodium 276 mg

Potassium 375mg

Protein 28.8 g

Jerk chicken

Preparation time: 10 minutes

Cooking time: 6 hours

Servings: 5

Ingredients

- 5 drumsticks and 5 wings
- 4 teaspoons of salt
- 4 teaspoons of paprika
- 1 teaspoon of cayenne pepper
- 2 teaspoons of onion powder
- 2 teaspoons of thyme
- 2 teaspoons of white pepper
- 2 teaspoons of garlic powder
- 1 teaspoon of black pepper

Directions:

1. Start by throwing all the Ingredients into the Slow cooker.
2. Cover it and cook for 6 hours on Low Settings.
3. Garnish as desired.
4. Serve warm.

Nutrition:

Calories 249

Total Fat 11.9 g

Saturated Fat 1.7 g

Cholesterol 78 mg

Total Carbs 1.8 g

Fiber 1.1 g

Sugar 0.3 g

Sodium 79 mg

Potassium 264 mg

Protein 35 g

CPSIA information can be obtained
at www.ICGtesting.com
Printed in the USA
BVHW052029120421
604748BV00001B/116

9 781801 831222